Modern Anesthesia And Hepatitis C

HALA GOMA

PROFESSOR OF ANESTHESIA CAIRO UNIVERSITY

Table of content

Introduction

- The main goal of the anesthesiologist is to avoid making the hepatic disease (with perhaps its
- metabolic and CNS toxicity) worse and increasing the chance of renal failure, coma, and death.
- All anesthetics tested (general, narcotic-nitrous oxide, and regional) have caused transient
- abnormalities in liver function test results. These abnormalities were magnified by upper intra-abdominal surgery and occurred regardless of preexisting liver disease.
- Patients whose preoperative liver function tests are abnormal will obviously have a higher
- Incidence of abnormal results on postoperative liver function test
- In addition to preexisting hepatic disease and the operative site, hypokalemia, hypotension, sepsis, and the need for blood transfusion
- All contribute to postoperative hepatic dysfunction. Thus, anesthesia and surgery probably exacerbate
- Hepatic disease and there by clearly increase morbidity and mortality.
- The liver performs many functions: it synthesizes substances (e.g., proteins, clotting factors), detoxifies the
- Body of both drugs and the products of normal human metabolism, excretes waste products, and
- Stores and supplies energy. Tests of liver functionassess synthesis (cholesterol levels, prothrombin

- time [PT], albumin levels), cellular integrity (aspartate aminotransferase [AST], alanine
- Aminotransferase [ALT], lactate dehydrogenase, alkaline phosphatase), the liver's ability to detoxify
- The body (e.g., ammonia, direct bilirubin, or lidocaine levels), and the liver's ability to excrete certain
- Substances (sulfobromophthalein retention, total bilirubin levels).
- In examining the effects of anesthesia (with or without surgery) on liver function and measures to
- Reduce risk in patients with preexisting liver disease, investigators have often looked at one or more of the aforementioned tests or, more commonly, at major end points of morbidity (jaundice) or mortality.

- Approximately 1 in 700 to 800
- Patients who are otherwise healthy and scheduled for surgery will have abnormal preoperative
- Results of liver function tests; of these patients, jaundice will develop in 1 in 3 .

- Now days with introduction of modern inhalational anesthestics ,as desflurane and sevoflurane with less hepatotoxicity.

- Desflurane is considered to be the safest inhalation anesthetic especially for patients who may have been sensitized by previous halothane exposure.
- Hepatotoxicity after halothane inhalation is common and has been studied extensively.1 In approximately 20% of patients given halothane anesthesia repeatedly, a mild hepatitis with

low-grade fever, nausea, and a mild transient elevation of liver enzymes is observed. In contrast, a fulminant hepatitis occurs in 1 of 20,000 patients exposed to halothane and is characterized by jaundice, hepatomegaly, hepatic encephalopathy, and markedly increased liver enzymes.

- Risk factors include obesity, female sex, middle age, and multiple anesthetics over a short period of time
- Current evidence suggests an immunologic basis for halothane hepatitis. Repeated halothane administrations increase the incidence of hepatitis complicated by fever, arthralgias, eosinophilia, and skin rashes.
- Halothane is metabolized by hepatic cytochrome P450 to trifluoroacetyl chloride, which covalently trifluoroacetylates several liver proteins in the endoplasmatic reticulum. Sera from patients suffering from halothane hepatitis often contain circulating antibodies directed against liver microsomal proteins that have been trifluoroacetylated by the reactive trifluoroacetyl chloride metabolite of halothane.
- The modified proteins are immunogenic in certain patients and may lead to the production of specific antibodies or even cytotoxic T cells, which may cause hepatic injury
- desflurane are metabolized by liver cytochrome P450 to acylated liver protein adducts by a mechanism similar to that of halothane.6 This raises the possibility that enflurane, isoflurane, and desflurane might cause hepatotoxicity by a mechanism similar to that of halothane, but at a lower incidence.
- This might be explained by the fact that the degree of oxidative biodegradation of these anesthetics appears to be highly variable with the degree of metabolism directly related to the potential for hepatic injury. Whereas 20% of administered halothane undergoes metabolism, Desflurane strongly resists biotransformation, with only 0.01% being

metabolized. it appears that even a very small amount of biotransformation

- Sevoflurane is a widely used major anesthetic agent with rapid onset of action and rapid dispersal.
- Because of its rapid onset of action and lack of irritability to the airways, sevoflurane can be used to both induce and maintain anesthesia.
- Sevoflurane became available for use in the United States in 1995.
- Sevoflurane must be administered in a controlled situation by a properly trained and credentialed anesthesiologist or nurse anesthetist and is typically given in concentrations of 2% to 4% with oxygen.

Hepatotoxicity

- Prospective, serial blood testing often demonstrates minor transient elevations in serum aminotransferase levels in the 1 to 2 weeks after major surgery.
- Appearance of ALT levels above 10 times the upper limit of normal, however, is distinctly unusual and points to significant hepatotoxicity.
- Clinically apparent, severe hepatic injury from sevoflurane is very rare
- A strong risk factor is previous exposure to any of the halogenated anesthetics and particularly a history of halothane hepatitis or unexplained fever and rash after anesthesia with one of these agents.
- The differential diagnosis of acute liver injury after surgery and anesthesia is sometimes difficult, and a clinical picture similar to sevoflurane induced hepatitis can be caused by

shock or ischemia, sepsis, other idiosyncratic forms of drug induced liver injury and acute viral or herpes hepatitis.

- The TFA adducts induce antibodies that can be detected in patients with sevoflurane- as well as halothane hepatotoxicity and are also found in a proportion of health care workers exposed to the volatile anesthetics.

Normal physiological functions of the liver:

1-Synthetic functions: .

- **Plasma proteins produced by hepatocytes include: albumin, fibrinogen, prothrombin, a-fetoprotein, a2-macroglobin, hemopexin, transferrin, complenent components C_3,C_6 andC_1, a_1-antitrypsin, caeruloplasmin.**
- **fetoprotein peaks about 16 weeks gestation and disappears a few weeks after birth. It may reappear in association with chronic hepatitis and a number of carcinomas**
- **macroglobin functions as a protease inhibitor. It is active in the inhibition of thrombin and plasmin.**
- **protein C, insulin-like growth factor,and other clotting factors.**

2-Clearance of damaged red blood cells & bacteria by phagocytosis

Kupffer cells are reticuloendothelial cells resident in the liver sinusoids that scavange damaged RBCs and bacteria. Kupffer cells lyse RBCs into heme and globin. Globin is further catabolized into polypeptide components for reuse. Heme is broken into biliverdin and iron. Biliverdin is converted to bilirubin. Iron is transported by transferrin to the liver and spleen for storage and to the bone for hematopoiesis.

3-Biotransformation of toxins, hormones, and drugs

There are many enzymes responsible for changing substance to be water soluble and excererted in urine and feces.there are 2 phases in this biotransformation .

Phase 1:

biotransformations the cytochrome P450 enzymes alter the target molecule by adding or exposing functional groups such as -OH or –COOH.

Phase 2:

Addition of sugars, amino acids, sulfates or acetyl groups to the functional group which makes them more water soluble by biotransformation enzymes.

Storage functions of the liver:

Vitamin A stores are concentrated in fat droplets within the stellate cells of the liver. Vitamin B12, Vitamin D stores equal about 3-4 months. Small amounts of Vitamins E and K and Vitamin C are stored in the liver.

Metabolic function of the liver:

Lipid metabolism:

Low density lipoproteins (LDL), high density lipoproteins (HDL) and fatty acids. Large lipoprotein molecules are broken into smaller units by the lytic action of lipoprotein lipase (LPL) expressed on endothelium of vessels. Circulating lipoproteins attach to receptors on the hepatocyte. This lipoprotein are held near the heptocyte surface and exposed to hepatic lipase compounds. Low Density Lipoprotein receptors transfer the lipoprotein by the process of endocytosis.

Carbohydrate metabolism:

There are three metabolic processes to manage carbohydrates to insure adequate blood glucose:

Glycogenesis –

Excess glucose, fructose, and galactose are converted to glycogen and stored in the liver.

Glycogenolysis –

when blood glucose falls, the liver breaks down stored glycogen to raise blood glucose levels.

Gluconeogenesis –

The liver can synthesize glucose from lactic acid, some amino acids and glycerol. When glucose is low, the metabolism of fatty acids can conserve available glucose.

Protein metabolism:

Oxidative deamination breaks amino acids into keto acid and an ammonia molecule. The keto acid is used in the Kreb's cycle to produce ATP. The liver combines ammonia with CO_2 to form urea and H_2O

Normal range of liver function according to mayo clinic:

- ALT. 7 to 55 units per liter (U/L)

- AST. 8 to 48 U/L

- ALP. 45 to 115 U/L

- Albumin. 3.5 to 5.0 grams per deciliter (g/dL)

- Total protein. 6.3 to 7.9 g/dL

- Bilirubin. 0.1 to 1.0 mg/dL

- GGT. 9 to 48 U/L

- **LD. 122 to 222 U/Lkkk**

PT. 9.5 to 13.8 seconds

HCV currently infects nearly 2% of the world's population. In Egypt the situation is very critical. Hepatitis C virus constitutes an epidemic in Egypt which is having the highest prevalence in the world. Nowhere else is there an HCV epidemic that affects a whole country. In all other countries, the prevalence of HCV is between 1% to 2%. There are a few exceptions where the prevalence of HCV is 3%. In Egypt however, the prevalence of HCV is 14.7%. Just about every family in Egypt is touched by hepatitis C. The blood borne virus, which is highly infectious, infects at least 1 in 10 of the population aged 15 to 59.

- There are seven major genotypes of HCV, which are indicated numerically from one to seven, The prevalent genotype in Egypt is type 4 (73%) followed by genotype 1 (26%), whereas mixed HCV genotypes infection was found in 15.7% in cases in Egypt.

Methods of Transmission:

1. Transfusion of blood contaminated with HCV was once an important source of transmission.

2. Persons who inject illegal drugs with nonsterile needles or who snort cocaine with shared straws are at highest risk for HCV infection. The

3.   most new HCV infections are related to intravenous drug abuse (IVDA).

4.   Transmission of HCV to health care workers may occur via needle-stick injuries or other occupational exposures. Needle-stick injuries in the health care setting result in a 3% risk of HCV transmission.

5.   Nosocomial patient-to-patient transmission may occur by means of a contaminated colonoscope, via dialysis, or during surgery, including organ transplantation before 1992.

6.   HCV may also be transmitted via tattooing, sharing razors, and acupuncture. The use of disposable needles for acupuncture, which has become standard practice in the United States, eliminates this transmission route.

7.   Coinfection with human immunodeficiency virus (HIV) type 1 appears to increase the risk of both sexual and maternal-fetal transmission of HCV.

8.   Casual household contact and contact with the saliva of those infected are inefficient modes of transmission. No risk factors are identified in approximately 10% of cases.

Clinical picture of hepatits C patient:

Most patients with acute and chronic infection are asymptomatic.

Acute HCV infection is usually subclinical: overt hepatitis develops in 10% of infected patient. Fulminant HCV is rare, but may occur more commonly in liver transplant recipients. The incubation period is around 7 weeks but can range from 2 to 12 weeks. Anorexia, myalgia and right upper quadrant pain may be present but are nonspecific.

Acute phase:

The period immediately following infection is called the 'acute phase'. This lasts about six months.

If the immune system does not manage to clear the virus in this time, the disease is considered to have moved into a long-term or 'chronic phase'.

Because of the damage it can cause to the liver, HCV is classified as a liver disease.

<u>Cirrhosis</u>

Compensated' the liver can continue to carry out most of its functions despite extensive scarring.

Decompensated'. If the liver's functions are seriously affected then this is called

The symptoms of this stage are:

- Portal Hypertension - when blood cannot properly flow through the liver and pressure rises in the portal vein leading into the liver.
- Variceal Bleeding - when the portal hypertension forces blood to re-route through veins that are too small and consequently burst, often in the oesophagus (between the throat and the stomach), causing potentially life-threatening internal bleeding. Oedema - when the liver stops producing enough albumin. This regulates the amount of fluid in cells.

<u>ascites'.</u>

- This fluid then builds up, typically in the stomach, and is known as '
- Hepatic Encephalopathy - when the liver stops properly filtering poisons and toxins. These then build up in the brain leading to serious mental confusion and sometimes coma.

  liver cancer.
- This can develop from either compensated or decompensated cirrhosis.

Factors affecting the progression of hepatitis C infection to cirrhosis

- Viral factors:
- Hepatitis C virus RNA load
- Genotype 1b
- **Host factors**

- Age at infection
- Male sex
- Nonwhite race
- Coinfection (hepatitis B virus, HIV-1)
- Comorbid disease (iron overload, nonalcoholic steatohepatitis)
- Genetic polymorphisms
- Disease expression (elevated levels of alanine aminotransferase, stage of fibrosis at diagnosis)

- Metabolic factors (obesity, insulin resistance, steatosis)
- Immunosuppression (organ transplantation)

- **Other factors**

- Alcohol (greater than 50 g/d)
- Smoking
- Environmental toxin

Extrahepatic manifestation of hepatitis C patients

Cardiovascular system

- Hyperdynamic circulation with a high cardiac output and low systemic vascular resistance.
- they have risk factors for coronary artery disease such as cigarette smoking and hyperlipidaemia.
- vasodilatation reduces left ventricular workload caused by cover underlying coronary artery disease and cardiomyopathy; these may become apparent during anaesthesia or surgery.

Respiratory

- Diaphragmatic splinting from ascites or
- Pleural effusions restricts alveolar ventilation,
- Reduces FRC,
- Atelectasis and hypoxia.
- Gastro-oesophageal reflux disease,

- Acute alcohol ingestion, and massive ascites may increase the risk of aspiration of gastric contents.
- Intrapulmonary arteriovenous shunting may also occur.
- Patients may experience dyspnoea and hypoxaemia when sitting upright, which improves on lying flat (orthodeoxia).

Hepatopulmonary syndrome

- The presence of pulmonary vascular shunting hypoxaemia may be severe which can be reversed by liver transplantation in suitable cases.
- pulmonary hypertension with increased pulmonary vascular resistance and normal pulmonary capillary wedge pressure.

- **Haematological**

Anaemia
Chronic illness
Calnutrition.

- Coagulopathy, particularly affecting the vitamin K-dependent factors II, VII, IX, and X.
- Thrombocytopaenia and platelet dysfunction are common.

Renal and metabolic

- Secondary hyperaldosteronism leads to water retention and hyponatraemia resulting in the formation of ascites and peripheral oedema.

- Loop diuretics used to treat the ascites and oedema can cause relative hypovolaemia and hypokalaemia.
- aldosterone antagonist spironoloactone can cause hyperkalaemia.
- Hepatorenal syndrome, caused by renal hypoperfusion, portal hypertension, intra-abdominal hypertension, and nephrotoxins alone or in combination.
- Vasodilatation associated with general anaesthesia may result in renal hypoperfusion and the development of pre-renal renal failure. Any acute deterioration in liver function

Central nervous system

- Hepatic encephalopathy in can be precipitated by infection, gasttrontestinal haemorrhage,
- Electrolyte or acid–base disturbance, sedative drugs,
- Hypoglycaemia, hypoxia, hypotension, or excessive dietary intake of protein.

Risk factors of morbidity and mortality of chronic liver cirrihosis:

1. **Type of surgery**
2. **Emergent Abdominal, especially cholecystectomy, gastric resection, or colectomy**
3. **Cardiac surgery.**

4. Hepatic resection

5. Characteristics of patient :

6. Portal hypertension

7. Child's class (C > B)

8. Ascites.

9. Encephalopathy .

10. Infection.

11. Anemia.

12. Malnutrition..

13. Jaundice .

14. Hypoalbuminemia .

15. Prolonged prothrombin time (>2.5 sec above control) that does not correct with vitamin K Abnormal quantitative liver function tests (*e.g.,* galactose elimination capacity, aminopyrine breath test, indocyanine green clearance, monoethylglycinexylidide test.

16. Hypoxemia.

EFFECTS OF ANESTHESIA AND SURGERY ON THE LIVER

- Anesthesia causes a moderate reduction in hepatic arterial blood flow and hepatic oxygen uptaE.

- the reduction in hepatic blood flow during the first 30 minutes of anesthesia averaged 35% among patients without liver disease liver blood flow returned to baseline during surgery,

- Either the initial hypoperfusion or reperfusion injury, or both, may contribute to postoperative liver dysfunction when it occurs.

- Patients with liver disease are more likely than patients without liver disease to experience hepatic decompensation with anesthesia.

- Effects of Hypercarbia: it initiates sympathetic stimulation of the splanchnic vasculature, thereby decreasing portal blood flow, and should be avoided in patients with liver disease. The pCO_2 should be

maintained in the range of 35 to 40 mm Hg during surgery.

Low Flow Anesthesia

Low flow anesthesia implies a carrier gas flow less than that attainable with a non-absorber breathing system.

Closed system anesthesia
Modern equipment permits the further reduction of the carrier gas flow to the ultimate degree of providing the patient's requirements .
 If nitrous oxide is not used, this gas need only comprise oxygen and air in the proportions required to provide an acceptable inspired oxygen concentration.
Modern inhalational anaesthetic agents are metabolized to a small extent only and are largely exhaled unchanged.

Characteristics of Low Flow Anaesthesia
- Increased rebreathing volume
- Less excess gas
- Difference of gas composition – Fresh gas versus gas in the circuit

Long time constants

Advantages of low flow techniques:
1. Economy: Significant savings can be achieved with lower flows of nitrous oxide and oxygen, but the greatest savings occurs with the potent volatile agents. These are partly offset by increased absorbent usage, but this cost is small.

2. Reduced Operating Room Pollution: With lower flows, there will be less anesthetic agent put into the operating room. However, the use of low-flow techniques does not eliminate the need for scavenging, because high flows are still necessary at times. Since less volatile agent is used, vaporizers have to be filled less frequently so that exposure to anesthetic vapors during filling is decreased.

- Reduced Environmental Pollution: Fluorocarbons and nitrous oxide attack the earth's ozone layer, and nitrous oxide contributes to the greenhouse effect.

Disadvantages of low flow techniques:

1. More Attention Required: With closed system anesthesia, fresh gas flow into the system must be kept in balance with uptake. This requires frequent adjustments.

2. Inability to Quickly Alter Inspired Concentrations: The use of low fresh gas flows prevents the rapid changes in fresh gas concentration in the breathing system that occurs with high gas flows. As a result, it may be more difficult to control acute hemodynamic responses. Danger of Hypercarbia: Hypercarbia resulting from exhausted absorbent, incompetent unidirectional valves or the absorber being left in the bypass position will be greater when low flows are used.

3. **<u>Accumulation of Undesirable Gases in the System:</u>**

a.   Carbon Monoxide: Carbon monoxide from the interaction of desiccated absorbent and anesthetic agent.

b.   Acetone, Methane, Hydrogen, and Ethanol Accumulation of acetone in blood during long-term anesthesia with closed systems.

c.   Compound A: It is accepted that prolonged sevoflurane anesthesia with low fresh gas flows results in proteinuria, glycosuria, and enzymuria. However, this is not, and has not been shown to be, associated with any clinical manifestations, even when such a technique is applied to patients with pre-existing biochemical renal abnormalities.

d.   Furthermore, it occurs if isoflurane is used in place of sevoflurane and seems also to be independent of carrier gas flow rate. The FDA recommended that sevoflurane not be used with fresh gas flows of less than 2 L/minute. This recommendation has been revised in 1997 to suggest that flow rates of 1 L/minute are acceptable but should not exceed 2 minimum alveolar concentrations (MAC)-hours. Some investigators feel that Compound A should not be a real clinical concern and that restricting the use of low fresh gas flows with sevoflurane cannot be justified

e.   Argon: If oxygen is supplied from an oxygen concentrator, there will be an accumulation of argon with low fresh gas flows.

f.   Nitrogen: with using oxygen/ nitrous mixtures Other: An acrylic monomer is exhaled when joint prostheses are surgically cemented. During this period, the system should be vented to prevent rebreathing of this chemical.

5.   Faster Absorbent Exhaustion: The lower the fresh gas flow, the faster the absorbent is exhausted

Requirements for the use of low flow techniques:
   <u>Monitoring</u>

- Hypoxia
- Gas volume deficiency
- Misdosage of volatiles
- Reduced controllability
- Exhaustion of the absorbent

<u>for Safe Performance of Low Flow Anaesthesia:</u>

Inspiratory oxygen concentration

Airway pressure and/or minute volume

Anaesthetic agent concentration in the circuit

Expiratory CO2-concentration

<u>The features of the anesthetic machine with respect to the fresh gas controls, the vaporisers, and the rebreathing system:</u>

- Fresh gas controls should work precisely
- flow meter tubes should be calibrated and graduated in the low flow range. Low and high flow rotameter tubes in tandem arrangement are advantageous.
- electronic fresh gas flow displays, allowing the setting of very low flows.
- The vaporizers should feature pressure-, temperature-, and flow compensation, a demand being met by all modern vaporizers.
- Using conventional anaesthetic machines with vaporizers outside the circuit, the limitation of the maximum output of the vaporizers at a concentration equalling 3-5 times the respective MAC makes it impossible to use anaesthetic agents with comparatively high solubility like halothane or enflurane in closed sytem anaesthesia.
- The leakage rate of the rebreathing systems must not exceed 100 mL/min at an internal system pressure of 20 mbar to meet the demands on gas tightness for performance of all different techniques of low flow anaesthesia.

- **Classification of anethesia methods using low fresh gas flow**

Low flow anaesthesia

It starts initially with high fresh gas flows between 4 L/min and 6 L/min and then reduced to 1.0 L/min after 10 min.

Minimal Flow anesthesia

- It starts with an initial phase of 15-20 min of 4-6 L/min, followed by a reduction of fresh gas flow down to 0.5 L/min.
- **Quantitative closed-loop anesthesia**.
- If fresh gas flow is continuously adjusted with a dosing apparatus to meet individual patient gas uptake and the amount of oxygen, nitrous oxide and inhalation anaesthetic is replaced, which is actually absorbed by the patient at any given time.
- (non-quantitative or nearly closed circuit anesthesia.
- It can also be performed by manually adjusting the fresh gas flow volume, without exact knowledge of the uptake of patient

Classification according to carrier gases

A) Oxygen as a carrier gas

High oxygen concentration in inhaled air

1. Increases patient safety,
2. Reduces the incidence of post-operative wound infections
3. Reduce the frequency of nausea and vomiting.
4. The increased likelihood of atelectasis at high oxygen tensions as compared to ventilation at lower oxygen concentrations appears to have no clinical effect on post-operative gas exchange or ventilation function.

5. The use of recruitment manoeuvres and positive end-expiratory pressures serve to inhibit atelectasis formation. Some contraindications exist for ventilation with high oxygen concentrations in patients with increased bronchial secretions; bronchioles may become clogged and are consecutively cut-off from ventilation.

Oxygen and medical air as a carrier gas mixture

- If the anesthesia machine is equipped with a gas dosing system designed for use with minimal flow anesthesia, the Anaesthetist can adjust the composition of the carrier gas mixture to achieve the desired oxygen concentration in the breathing circuit.
- Economical anesthesia, closed loop anesthesia, is possible.
- If the anesthesia machine uses a dosing apparatus, which does not allow low levels of gas flow for medical air.
- the anesthetist must then decide whether he or she is willing to do without the economic advantages of low or minimal flow anesthesia and instead use low inspiratory oxygen concentrations during anesthesia.
- Such machines can, however, be used to perform closed-loop anesthesia, which substitutes small amounts of pure oxygen following an initial high flow phase.

- If medical air is not available or the anaesthesia machine is not equipped with a corresponding dosing apparatus, the only possible alternative is to avoid the use of nitrous oxide and use pure oxygen as the carrier gas as described above.

B) Low flow anaesthesia using an oxygen/nitrous oxide carrier gas

- Induction of low flow anesthesia is identical to conventional methods: Following pre-oxygenation, injection of an opioid and hypnotic agent and if desired, a muscle relaxant, an endotracheal tube or laryngeal mask is placed in position.
- Patient is connected to the rebreathing system.
- With the connection of the patient to the anaesthesia machine, an initial phase of high fresh gas flow (4-6 L/min) follows.
- During this initial phase, adequate denitrogenation and distribution of anaesthetic gases in the desired concentration throughout the system is achieved and the desired level of anaesthesia is attained.
- The duration of the initial phase is determined by the amount of flow reduction and the individual gas uptake (4-5 L/min, 6-8 min).
- After this time, oxygen and nitrous oxide levels reach 30% O_2 and 65% N_2O, respectively.
- sevoflurane require 2.5% setting

- Desflurane requires a 4-6% setting. After 6-8 min, an expiratory concentration corresponding to 0.8 minimum alveolar concentration (MAC) of the respective anesthetic agent is attained.
- At an additive nitrous oxide concentration of 50-60%, this value approximately corresponds to AD_{95}, or the anesthetic agent concentration at which 95% of patients tolerate a skin incision without noticeable reaction.

Sevoflurane & Desflurane use with low flow techniques:

- Both inhalation anesthetics are characterised by low solubility, correspondingly low individual uptake, and comparatively low anesthetic potency.
- the maximum output of both of the vaporisers is limited to a fairly high concentration, 8.0 vol% for sevoflurane, and 18.0 vol% for desflurane.
- if the flow is kept as low as 0.5 L/min, the amount of vapour delivered into the system reaches 43.5 mL/min with sevoflurane or even 110 mL/min with desflurane at its maximum.
- According to Conway's formula. $T = V_S/(V_F - V_U)$ the time constant T is proportional to the system volume V_S (machine and lung volume) and at a constant rate of uptake V_U, inversely proportional to the amount of anesthetic agent fed into the system at the time.

- low individual uptake together with high amount of agent delivered into the breathing system results in a marked decrease of the time constant.
- Thus, even if the flow is kept unchanged at a very low flow rate, a comparatively rapid increase of the agent's concentration can be gained when use is made of the maximum output of the vaporizer. The use of Desflurane will result in an even more pronounced decrease of the time constant than the use of Sevoflurane.

References

1. Amer FA, Gohar M, Yousef M. Epidemiology of Hepatitis C Virus Infection in Egypt; 2015; IJTDH, 7(3): 119-131.

2. Xu LZ, Larzul D, Delaporte E, Bréchot C, Kremsdorf D. Hepatitis C virus genotype 4 128 is highly prevalent in central Africa (Gabon). J Gen Virol. 1994;75(9):2393–2398

3. Stramer SL, Glynn SA, Kleinman SH, Strong DM, Caglioti S, Wright DJ, Dodd RY, Busch MP. Detection of HIV-1 and HCV infections among antibody-negative blood donors by nucleic acid–amplification testing. New England Journal of Medicine. 2004 Aug. 351(8):760-8.

4. Rischitelli G, Harris J, McCauley L, Gershon R, Guidotti T. The risk of acquiring hepatitis B or C among public safety workers: a systematic review. *Am J Prev Med*. 2001 May. 20(4):299-306

5. Yeung LT, King SM, Roberts EA. Mother-to-infant transmission of hepatitis C virus. *Hepatology*. 2001 Aug. 34(2):223-9

6. Sultan MT, Rahman MM, Begum S. Epidemiology of hepatitis C virus (HCV) infection. Journal of Bangladesh College of Physicians and Surgeons. 2009;27(3):160-5.

7. Patel K, Muir AJ, McHutchison JG. Diagnosis and treatment of chronic hepatitis C infection. British Medical Journal. 2006 Apr; 332(7548):1013-7.

8. Strunin L, Eagle CJ. Hepatic diseases. In: Benumof JL, editor. Anesthesia & Uncommon Diseases. 4th

Edn. Philadelphia: WB Saunders Company;1998. p.147-74.

9. Wiklund RA. Preoperative preparation of patients with advanced liver disease.Crit Care Med 2004;32:S106-15.

10. Vaja R, McNicol L, Sisley I. Anaesthesia for patients with liver disease. Continuing Education in Anaesthesia, Critical Care & Pain. 2010 Feb 1;10(1):15-9.

11. Wiklund RA. Preoperative preparation of patients with advanced liver disease.Crit Care Med 2004;32:S106-15.

12. Budhiraja R, Hassoun P., Portopulmonary hypertension: a tale of two circulations. Chest 2003; 123:562-76.

13. Wiklund RA. Preoperative preparation of patients with advanced liver disease.Crit Care Med 2004;32:S106-15.

14. Cade R, Wagemaker H, Vogel S, Mars D, Hood-Lewis D, Privette M, Peterson J, Schlein E, Hawkins R, Raulerson D, Campbell K. Hepatorenal syndrome. Studies of the effect of vascular volume and intraperitoneal pressure on renal and hepatic function. The American journal of medicine. 1987 Mar 31;82:427-38.

15. Strunin L, Eagle CJ. Hepatic diseases. In: Benumof JL, editor. Anesthesia & Uncommon Diseases. 4th Edn. Philadelphia: WB Saunders Company; 1998. p.147-74.

16. DeRitis F, Coltori M, Gisuti G. Serum transaminase activities in liver disease. Lancet. 1972;1:685–87.

17. Cassidy WM, Reynolds TB. Serum lactic dehydrogenase in the differential diagnosis of acute hepatocellular injury. Journal of clinical gastroenterology. 1994 Sep 1;19(2):118-21.

18. [Guideline] Garcia J. Hepatitis C: USPSTF recommends all baby boomers be screened. Medscape Medical News from WebMD. Available at http://www.medscape.com/viewarticle/806836. Jun 24 2013; Accessed: Jun 26 2013.

19. Eger E. Low Flow Anaesthesia: The Theory and Practice of Low Flow, Minimal Flow and Closed System Anaesthesia. The Journal of the American Society of Anesthesiologists. 2002 Aug 1;97(2):530-.

20. De Cooman S, Lecain A, Sosnowski M, De Wolf AM, Hendrickx JF. Desflurane consumption with the Zeus (R) during automated closed circuit versus low flow anesthesia. Acta Anæsthesiologica Belgica. 2009;60:35–7.[PubMed]

21. Baum JA. The carrier gas in anaesthesia: Nitrous oxide/oxygen, medical air/oxygen and pure oxygen.Curr Opin Anaesthesiol. 2004;17:513–6. [PubMed]

22. Hönemann C, Hagemann O, Doll D. Inhalational anaesthesia with low fresh gas flow. Indian journal of anaesthesia. 2013 Jul;57(4):34

23. Hönemann CW, Hahnenkamp K, Möllhoff T, Baum JA. Minimal-flow anaesthesia with controlled ventilation:

Comparison between laryngeal mask airway and endotracheal tube. Eur J Anaesthesiol.2001;18:458–66. [PubMed]

24. Hönemann CW, Hahnenkamp K, Möllhoff T, Baum JA. Minimal-flow anaesthesia with controlled ventilation: Comparison between laryngeal mask airway and endotracheal tube. Eur J Anaesthesiol.2001;18:458–66. [PubMed]

25. Hönemann C, Hagemann O, Doll D. Inhalational anaesthesia with low fresh gas flow. Indian journal of anaesthesia. 2013 Jul;57(4):345.

26. Eger E. Low Flow Anaesthesia: The Theory and Practice of Low Flow, Minimal Flow and Closed System Anaesthesia. The Journal of the American Society of Anesthesiologists. 2002 Aug 1;97(2):530-.

27. Bengtson JP, Sonander H, Stenqvist O. Comparison of costs of different anaesthetic techniques. Acta Anaesthesiol Scand 1988; 32: 33–3

28. Awati MN, Patil GA, Fathima A. KEYWORDS: Low flow anaesthesia, closed system anaesthesia, inhalational anaesthetics. LOW-FLOW ANAESTHESIA. 2014 Oct 20(237).

29. Logan M, Farmer JG. Anesthesia and the ozone layer. Br J Anaesth 1989; 63: 645–647., Sherman SJ, Cullen BF. Nitrous oxide and the greenhouse effect. Anesthesiology 1988; 68: 816–817.

30. Biro P. A formula to calculate oxygen uptake during low flow anesthesia based on FIO2 measurement. J Clin Monit Comput 1998; 14: 141–144.

31. Awati MN, Patil GA, Fathima A. KEYWORDS: Low flow anaesthesia, closed system anaesthesia, inhalational anaesthetics. LOW-FLOW ANAESTHESIA. 2014 Oct 20(237).

32. Kleeman PP. Humidity of anaesthetic gases with respect to low flow anaesthesia. Anaesth Intens Care 1994; 22: 396–408.

33. GA, Fathima A. KEYWORDS: Low flow anaesthesia, closed system anaesthesia, inhalational anaesthetics. LOW-FLOW ANAESTHESIA. 2014 Oct 20(237).

34. Avramov M, Griffin J, White P. The effect of fresh gas flow and anesthetic technique on the ability to control acute hemodynamic responses during surgery. Anesth Analg 1998; 87: 666–670.

35. Coppens MJ, Versichelen LFM, Rolly G, et al. The mechanisms of carbon monoxide production by inhalational agents. Anaesthesia 2006; 61: 462–468.

36. Tolly G, Versichelen LF, Mortier E. Methane accumulation during closed-circuit anesthesia. Anesth Analg 1994; 79: 545–547.

37. . Ebert T, Frink E, and Kharasch E Absence of biochemical evidence for renal and hepatic dysfunction after 8 hours of 1.25 MAC sevoflurane anaesthesia in volunteers. Anesthesiology 1998; 88: 601-10.

38. Parker CJR, Snowdon SL. Predicted and measured oxygen concentrations in the circle system using low fresh gas flows with oxygen supplied by an oxygen concentrator. Br J Anaesth 1988; 61: 397–402.

39. Philip JH. Closed circuit anesthesia. In: Ehrenwerth J, Eisenkraft JB, eds. Anesthesia Equipment, Principles and Applications. St. Louis: Mosby, 1993: 617–635.

40. . M. N. Awati, Gurulingappa A. Patil, Ahmedi Fathima, Samudyatha T. J. "Low Flow Anaesthesia". Journal of Evidence Based Medicine and Healthcare; Volume 1, Issue 9, October 31, 2014; Page: 1150-1162.

·

·

www.ingramcontent.com/pod-product-compliance
Lightning Source LLC
Chambersburg PA
CBHW070422190526
45169CB00003B/1368